Longevity Training-Book 6-Energy Body Health

This book is a transcription and reproduction of the training course materials from Course #6 "Energy Body Health"

The Energy Body is described by the Indians as consisting of the "Chakras" and the Chinese as being "The Energy Meridians".

You can learn to utilize and see this energy body to improve your health and longevity.

In this book we explore some details of the Energy Body and provide lots of exercises on how to move the energies around your physical body.

I learned about the Energy Body as a young man in college and learned how to take vital forces energy into my body which has had lots of benefits for me in the long run.

Longevity Training-Book 6-Energy Body Health

Longevity Training-Book 6-Energy Body Health

Copyright Page

The book is copyrighted for 2018

Longevity Training-Book 6-Energy Body Health

By Martin K. Ettington

ISBN: 9781792057137

Longevity Training-Book 6-Energy Body Health

Longevity Training-Book 6-Energy Body Health

Other books by Martin K. Ettington

Spiritual and Metaphysics Books:
Prophecy: A History and How to Guide
God Like Powers and Abilities
Enlightenment for Newbies
Removing Illusions to Find True
    Happiness
Using the Scientific Method to Study
    the Paranormal
A Compendium of Metaphysics and
    How to Guides (Six books
    together in one volume)
Love from the Heart
The Enlightenment Experience
Learn Your Soul's Purpose
Pursuing Enlightenment
A Modern Man's Search for Truth
Use Intuition and Prophecy to Improve
    Your Life
The Handbook of Spiritual and Energy
    Healing

Longevity & Immortality:
Physical Immortality: A History and
    How to Guide
The Commentaries of Living Immortals
Records of Extremely Long Lived
    Persons
Enlightenment and Immortality
Longevity Improvements from Science
The 10 Principles of Personal
    Longevity
Telomeres & Longevity
The Diets and Lifestyles of the Worlds
    Oldest Peoples
The Longevity Six Books Bundle

Science Fiction:
Out of This Universe
Personal Freedom-Parts 1 & 2
The Psychic Soldier Series:
    Book 1-Himalayan Journey
    Book 2-A Soldier is Born
    Book 3-Fighting For Right
    Book 4-Earth Protector
The Immortality Sci Fi Bundle

The God Like Powers Series:
Human Invisibility
Invulnerability and Shielding
Teleportation
Psychokinesis
Our Energy Body, Auras, and
Thoughtforms

The God Like Powers Series—
    Volume 1 Compilation

The Yoga Discovery Series:
Yoga-An Ancient Art Form
Hatha Yoga-Helping you Live Better
Raja Yoga-Through the Ages
The Yoga Discovery Package

Business & Coaching Books:
Creating, Paublishing, & Marketing
    Practitioner Ebooks
Building a Successful Longevity
    Coaching Business
Why Become a Coach?
The Professional Coaching Success
Trilogy
2020-Make Money Writing and Selling
    Books
The 2020 Handbook of High Paying
    Work Without a College Degree

Science, Technology, and Misc.
Future Predictions By and Engineer &
    Seer
The Unusual Science & Technology
    Bundle
The Real Atlantis-In the Eye of the
    Sahara
Are Cryptozoological Animals Real or
    Imaginary?
Real Time Travel Stories From a
    Psychic Engineer
Removing Limits On Our
    Consciousness-And
    Thinking Outside the Box
33 Incredible True Survival Stories
How to Survive Anything: From the
    Wilderness to Man Made
    Disasters
All About Mars Journeys and
    Settlement
Mining the Asteroid Belt

Ancient History
The Real Atlantis-In the Eye of the
Sahara
Ancient & Prehistoric Civilizations
Ancient & Prehistoric Civilizations-Book
    Two
The History of Antediluvian Giants
The Antediluvian History of Earth
Ancient Underground Cities and
    Tunnels
Strange Objects Which Should Not Exist
Strange and Ancient Places in the USA
A Theory of Ancient Prehistory And
    Giant Aliens
Aliens and Space

Longevity Training-Book 6-Energy Body Health

Aliens and Secret Technology
Aliens Are Already Among Us
Designing and Building Space Colonies
Humanity and the Universe
All About Moon Bases
All About Mars Journeys and Settlement

The Space and Aliens Six Books Bundle
A Theory of Ancient Prehistory and
  Giant Aliens
The Space Colonies and Space
  Structures Coloring Book
All About Asteroids

<u>The Longevity Training Series</u>

(A transcription of the online Multimedia Longevity Coaching Training Program)

The Personal Longevity Training Series-Book1-Long Lived Persons
The Personal Longevity Training Series-Book2-Your Soul's Purpose
The Personal Longevity Training Series-Book3-Enable Your Life Urge
The Personal Longevity Training Series-Book4-Your Spiritual Connection
The Personal Longevity Training Series-Book5-Having Love in Your Heart
The Personal Longevity Training Series-Book6-Energy Body Health
The Personal Longevity Training Series-Book7-The Science of Longevity
The Personal Longevity Training Series-Book8-Physical Body Health
The Personal Longevity Training Series-Book9-Avoiding Accidents
The Personal Longevity Training Series-Book10-Implementing These Principles

The Personal Longevity Training Series-Books One Thru Ten

These books are all available in digital and printed formats from my
website and on Amazon, Barnes & Noble, Apple ITunes, and many other sites

My Books Website is: http://mkettingtonbooks.com

Longevity Training-Book 6-Energy Body Health

<u>Signup for our Mailing List to get the following:</u>

1) A discount coupon for 25% discount on all books on our site

2) Occasional Notices of new books available

3) Occasional Email on other offerings of ours (Monthly)

Go to this link to sign-up:

http://personal-longevity.com/mkebooks/emailsignup/

And click this link to get the FREE 102 page Ebook titled "Secrets of Many Things"

If you have any questions about this book or other subjects please contact the Author at:

mke@mkettingtonbooks.com

Longevity Training-Book 6-Energy Body Health

Longevity Training-Book 6-Energy Body Health

Table of Contents

Longevity Training-Book 6-Energy Body Health

1.0 Introduction

Back in 2008 I became very interested in the field of Longevity and Physical Immortality. After a lot of research this led me to my first book on the subject "Physical Immortality: A History and How to Guide". This book was pretty popular and I wanted to continue learning about Longevity and what things we could do about it in our lives.

The subject continued to fascinate me to the point that I developed a Longevity Coaching program over a couple of years starting in 2011. This online training program was multimedia—consisting of videos, my writings on longevity to read, online exercises, and tests for each of ten courses. It also included a lot of additional resources for each course including extra courses on how to become a successful Longevity Coach. A student who completed the training and tests successfully would become certified as a "Longevity Coach" and authorized to teach this material to others.

I developed a set of ten principles on longevity which are as follows:

The 10 Principles of Personal Longevity are:

- The Reality of Long Lived People
- Defining Your Purpose in Life
- Enabling the Life Urge
- Your Spiritual Health
- Having Love in Your Heart
- Energy Body Health
- The Science of Longevity
- Physical Body Health
- Using your Intuition for Safety

- Implementation of these principles

What are the 10 Principles all about?

The Reality of Long Lived People

The first principle is where I provide lots of evidence of people who have lived well over the age of 120 years old to 150-180-200, and even a 256 year old man from China:

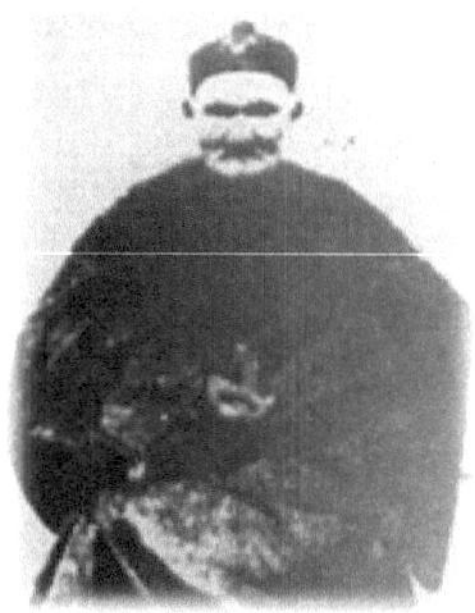

LI CHING-YUN: The Longest Lived person of record-256 Years (Source-The New York Times-May 6, 1933)

The Second Principle of Life Purpose

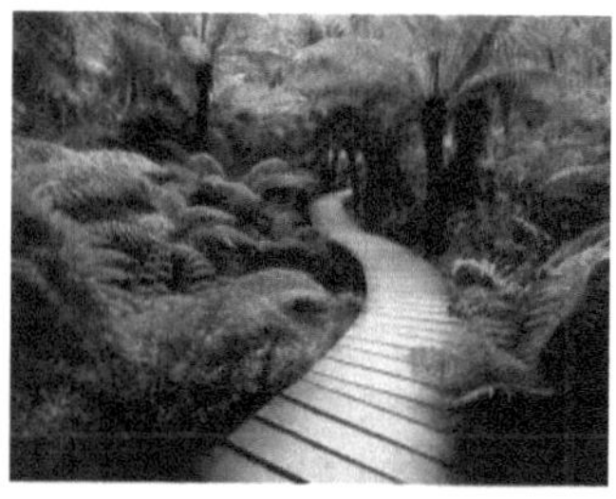

One of the things that occurred to me when I was putting the 10 principles together was that if one doesn't have a reason to live, or purpose in life--then what is the point?

This meant I had to add a very important step of how you can develop your own life purpose, or bring it up to date with your phase in life. Without reviewing your purpose-- then none of the rest of the principles matter.

Enabling the Life Urge

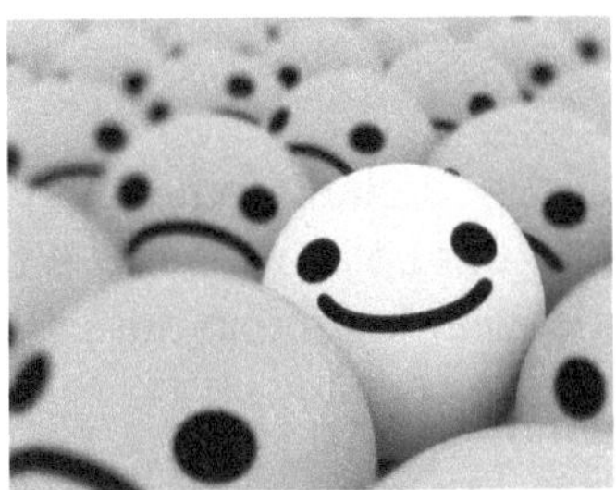

Have you ever realized how we are all programmed to expect to live through certain stages in life and then die?

It's so common in our society that we don't think it odd that we expect to die at a certain age?

Have you ever heard radio ads saying "You are getting up in your sixties and seventies" so it's time to come out to our cemetery and buy a plot"

How ridiculous is this? And do you see how much our subconscious has been programmed towards death?

This principle is all about reprogramming ourselves to have a more positive outlook on life and its possibilities.

Having a Spiritual Connection in Your Life

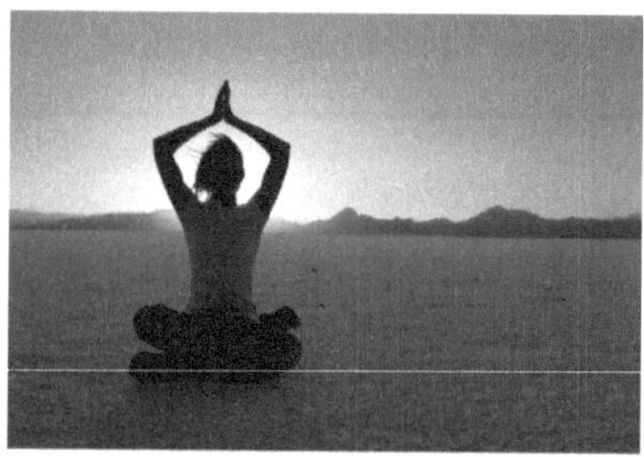

Most of us innately understand that we have a spiritual core in the center of our being. It is this spiritual core that we need to connect with to enable our physical health too.

It doesn't matter what religion you are. Regular meditation, deep prayer, or just walking in the woods helps you make and keep that connection in your life.

Having Love in Your Heart

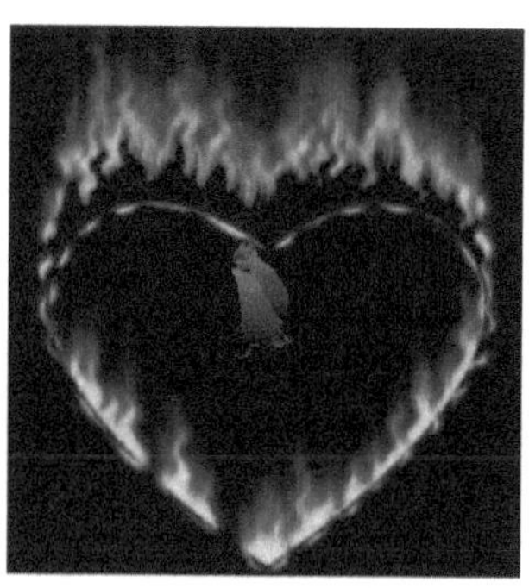

One of the most important things I learned in the last five years was that Unconditional Love is a real and physical thing. It is a powerful energy force in life and not just a philosophical belief system.

I considered it so important that I added it as a separate principle of longevity.

True Unconditional Love is healing, embodies happiness, and is a powerful part of our vital forces.

Energy Body Health

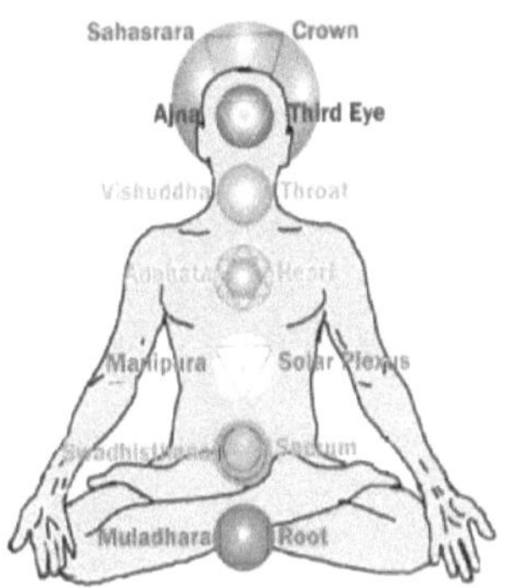

We all have an energy body which is part of our vital forces. The Indians talk about the "Chakras" and the Chinese talk about "Energy Meridians" in Acupuncture.

We should all learn different practices to keep our vital forces flowing for maximum health and vitality.

The Science of Longevity

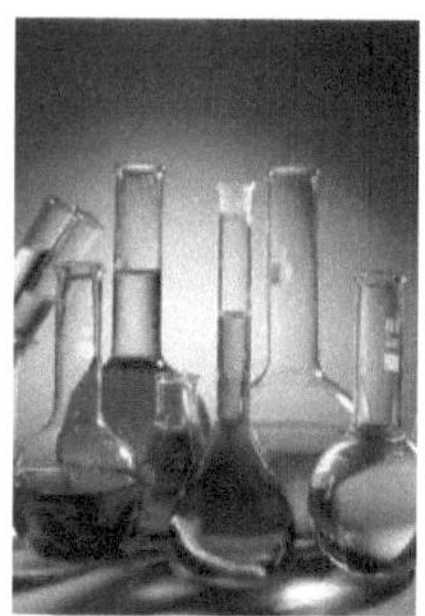

 Science and Medicine are making new discoveries all the time that we can take advantage of to extend our lives.

Why not take advantage of these discoveries which provide new therapies and supplements to increase our longevity.

There is also a lot we can learn from plants and animals. We all share the same genetic basis.

Some of these plants and animals live thousands of years and some cells are immortal.

What can we learn from them to apply to our lives?

Physical Body Health

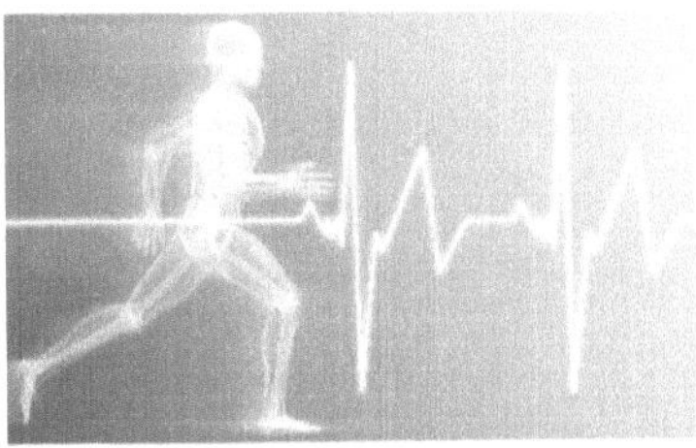

There are many types of supplements used for anti-aging for thousands of years. What can we learn about them that we can apply to our lives?

What other considerations about our physical health does nontraditional or alternative medicine offer?

Using Your Intuition for Safety

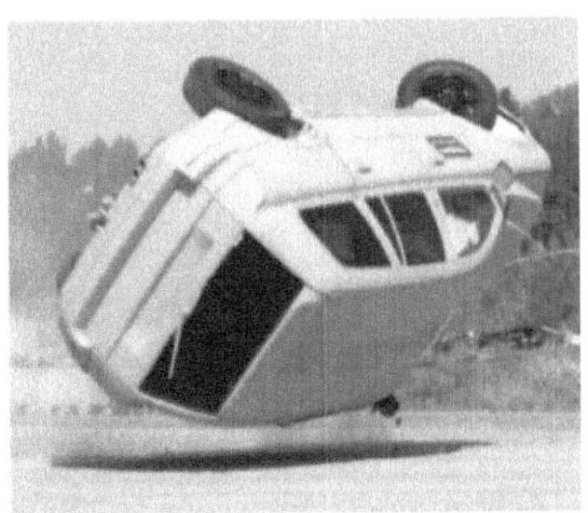

Once you have established your own long term health then what is the greatest danger you face?

ACCIDENTS

We can learn to use our intuition to make us safer as well as see potential future events which may be good too.

Why not open up to the possibilities of how our spirit has this natural ability in all of us?

Implementing These Principles in Your Life

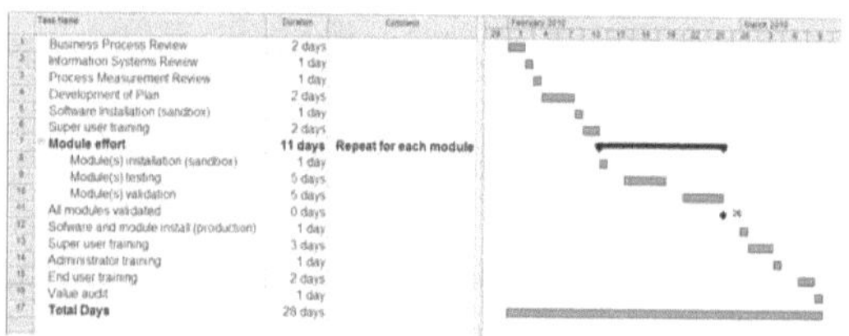

It's nice to read about all these concepts, but how can you really apply them to your own life?

This is what the chapter on implementation is all about, and it helps you plan a lifelong change in your health focus to live these principles and truly experience long term health, greater happiness, and extended longevity.

For five years I amended and improved these materials which now include a lot more information and helpful concepts for students wanting to improve their longevity and those of others.

I transcribed my videos and other materials to this book so you can read it all, and later hear it in an AudioBook.

This book is priced pretty inexpensively, compared to the online training and certification program which sells in total for $1,995 USD. If you are interested in taking the entire online program at a major discount, then please contact me at:

Marty@personal-longevity.com

Hope you enjoy these materials since when applied correctly they will significantly change your life.

2.0 PLP Concepts Overview

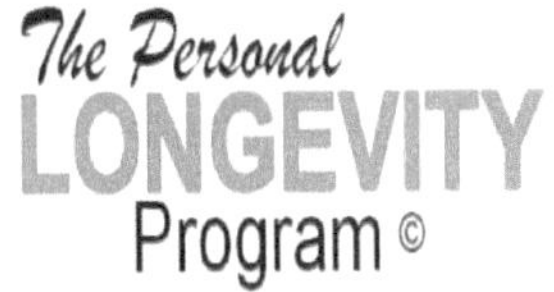

(Transcription of overview video)

Hello I'm Martin Ettington and I'd like to introduce you to the Personal Longevity Program which is an integrated holistic approach to long-term health. In this video we will only cover the high level concepts which comprise individual courses in the coaching certificate program for personal longevity.

The first concept is that long lived people exist and have existed for hundreds of thousands of years. We cover in the first course all about their records; along with people not only in places you might think like India, but in Europe and the United States-people who've lived long lives and well documented cases.

We discuss people who have lived well over the age of 120 and even the case of a Chinaman who lived to 256 years old. Plus a lot of mythology about people who have lived even longer lives so you get an idea that extending your life much longer than we think is currently medically and scientifically possible is certainly something that can happen.

The second course's concept has to do with finding your souls purpose. The point of wanting to live a long life is to know what your purpose in life is, so we go through some readings and some exercises to help you determine where soul's purpose in life is. Then doing goals as a fundamental concept so you will know the motivations in your life.

Third is the "Psychology of Living" also known by certain practitioners as "Removing the death Urge". The psychology of living has to do with seeking a positive image about your ability to live a long time. We tend to be programmed from birth about the idea that we are going to go through certain stages in our life as a child, as a teenager, and as adults. It's about reprogramming your subconscious as to the possibilities of a long life.

I've also learned in my life that it is very important to be able open your heart to unconditional love. When you're able to love unconditionally it also helps increase the strength of your immune system and fight off disease. So this is an aspect of spiritual growth. The courses also cover unconditional love and energy body forces. Managing your energy body is an important component of who you are in having energy working properly in your body and is another aspect of health for the length of longevity.

There are many types of scientific and medical research which are being done today and which will contribute to human longevity in the future.

Do you know that the average lifespan in the United States in 1900 was only about 40 years? We have doubled lifespan in the last century with current technologies but things under way in terms of scientific and medical improvements will help extend your lives further.

Also in this course on longevity we will cover a lot of the concepts which are being researched by scientists today. There are suggestions for more things you can do to do to use this science to improve your health along with physical supplements.

A unique thing that I thought about and decided to offer in these courses has to do with all my experiences in prophecy and how I was able to change outcomes on accidents that would occur to me by using simple exercises you can learn to change these outcomes. If you're in great health often the biggest thing you have to worry about are accidents.

We also provide guidelines you can follow on a daily basis and plans you can make to live healthier and happier and have a much longer life than you ever thought possible.

Thank you for listening !

3.0 Course #6 Intro Video

(Transcription of Video)

Hello I'm Marty Ettington. I'd like to welcome you to the personal longevity program's course number six on energy body health. This course is going to be all about the historical roots of the energy body. What it's about and talking about exercises to learn to use the energy body.

First of all in in terms of the historical roots of knowing about the existence of the energy body there are several cultures we can look at who learned about it thousands of years ago. But probably the best-known one is the Indian culture in India where the meditators and gurus learned about the chakra system and the energy pathways in the body. The chakras being different points throughout the body like the head, the heart, and the root of the spine where you can learn to open these energy centers to take in and manipulate energies throughout your body.

Similarly the Chinese also learned about the energy body. They mapped the energy meridians running throughout the body, and this is the basis for the medical practice called acupuncture. The Chinese have also known about the energy body for a couple thousand years at least. Other cultures are aware of the energy body too like if you've ever read Carlos Castaneda and his sorcerer teacher Don Juan who is a Mexican Yaqui Indian. Yaquis believed in learning to see the different energy fields that made all of us up and seeing each of us as a node in the in the underlying energy or spirit consciousness of the universe.

And also Patanjali the famous writer of the "Yoga Sutras of Patanjali" which I think is a very good scientific basis for the structure of consciousness and enlightenment. He talked about the many different levels of consciousness. You could call some of those levels of the energy body. Different authors and writers disagree on the levels and the energy body and many different levels of consciousness.

What they all agree about though is that there are specific layers of these core spirit levels of consciousness and energy. And then the physical body generally people who are energy practitioners believe that many diseases are caused by the energy system being clogged. For instance if your heart chakra is clogged for a long period of time that may give you heart problems. And I've actually talked to people who by doing energy work on their hearts were able to help healthier hearts.

So learning how to keep your energy system open and flowing is a key to long-term health. I want to talk about a couple of my experiences with energy body practices when I was nineteen. And first learning meditation-I learned from a blind middle-aged physicist named Sam Lentine who also told taught me at the same time how to open my Crown Chakra on the top of my head. And this was a revelatory experience because not only did I learn how to meditate and get to a very deeply relaxed state but I actually started to feel energy coming in through my Crown Chakra.

Ever since I've been nineteen I have been able to take in energy to revitalize me when I needed it. And also to learn how to do healing techniques. So it's very powerful to have your Crown Chakra open. And you can really feel the sensations. More recently in the last couple of years I did a lot of exercises to open my heart chakra. And the heart chakra is a whole different experience whereas the crown chakra is more intellectual and purely spiritual. The heart chakra is if anything more powerful. You feel its heat in your chest. Its love changes your whole attitude about relationships with people and the world around you. And I'm still evolving from that but I can tell you that that's also a very powerful experience. Other chakras can have powerful experiences on your body. And in your psyche too.

But this is just two of the stranger experiences which had made a major difference in my life. In fact the reason that I put in one of the courses in this course sequence on unconditional love is specifically because of my experiences with the Heart Chakra. I had known intellectually that was important before, but when my Heart Chakra actually opened and I was able to actually feel the power of all that God energy-that God love. I realize that it's also extremely important to your happiness and your health, so in the course you will also you'll find different types of exercises as well as books to read about the energy body, and the auras, and thought forms.

And also there's a couple of good exercises which are in videos you can watch. One is about cell regeneration, the other about sacred fire. These are both exercises that I practice quite a bit and I'll tell you a funny story about the cell regeneration one.

I had read that in another book-I think it was "Star Signs" and when I first tried it out the writer had said that people may smell of old leather old shoes about you which is the cells in your body releasing toxins. So I tried this out the first night after I'd read it and it was very powerful I had a lot of good feelings from it. And then in the morning when I was taking my son to school he said I smelled funny. I said what are you talking about he said-yeah you smell like old leather or old shoes. And I said "oh really?". So maybe there was something to it. I mean-I did get a good feeling from it but it seems like maybe it was really releasing the toxins in my body.

Sacred fire is also a very powerful purification visualization that helps you purify your body. In the energies in it-again through a visualization process-so there's additional resources in this course. Again to teach you more about the aura, to teach you about thoughtforms, and some presentations on the energy body. There's plenty to learn on the energy body. There's many techniques you can learn such as Tai Chi and Qigong just to name a couple out of many processes and techniques you can learn to enhance your energy body. And I strongly encourage it since this is one of the basis for long-term health and longevity. Thank you for listening and enjoy the course.

4.0 The Energy Body

1.0   The Importance of the Energy Body

Learning about the Aura, Chakras, and the Energy Body was the beginning of my serious education on the spiritual and paranormal.

I will in college at Rensselaer Polytechnic Institute in 1974 when I met Sam Lentine—a blind middle aged Physics PHD student who was also a strong clairvoyant and well developed psychic,

We became friends and I helped him develop a psychic development class where I first learned meditation and how to open my crown chakra to take in vital force energies.

This was an amazing experience because I learned about vital forces from first hand experiences which couldn't be denied by my analytical side.

If I hadn't learned about the energy body and how it works, then I think I would have been caught in the spiritual development slow lane for many decades.

Today, my crown chakra is open almost all the time with lots of energy coming in and it makes a big difference in my life.

*****

Whenever somebody talks about psychic or paranormal phenomena, the subject usually comes up about the aura, the energy body, chakras, and other related structures in the human body.

The problem is that western science does not officially recognize the existence of the energy body because of unreliable measurements and lack of acceptance of this part of our being.

Paintings of Auras exist going back hundreds and thousands of years, as do writings about the energy body.

Acupuncture has been practiced for thousands of years in China, and is generally accepted as having benefits in the west—even though a theory properly explaining how it works in conventional scientific terms doesn't exist.

I've written a number of books on the Spiritual and Paranormal, and realize that many people do not even accept the existence of this energy body-which hurts my credibility with those persons.

It's unfortunate that so many don't believe in the energy body, because understanding what the energy body is and how it works is the key to a focused approach of spiritual and psychic development.

2.0   The Human Aura in History

References to the aura can be traced back to the very beginnings of civilization. In the West we are likely most familiar with the aura as a glowing light or halo surrounding the heads of Jesus, Mary and saints in religious art. The aura denoted spiritual energy long before its depiction as halos in Christianity, however.

Ancient Egyptian art is full of representations of the aura. The Ancient Egyptians depicted halos around the heads of pharaohs and other important personages as well as deities.

The Ancient Greeks and Romans seem to have adopted the iconography and the head halo is still with us in Christianity. In India, the Hindu religion honor deities in the same manner.

Energy as the basis for life is at the core of Eastern religions; in China this energy is called "Chi," in India, it's referred to as "Prana." In mystical Hindu writings one finds reference to the "thousand-petaled lotus of light" surrounding the head of those who achieved enlightenment. (Walker, 373) (1)

One finds numerous allusions to visions of light and to light as the source of life in literature as well. One of the earliest written examples comes from the writings of Hildegard von Bingen (1098 - 1179), who produced major visionary and theological writings over the course of her lifetime. She describes in her writings her visions of luminous objects, as well as other visionary experiences of light. She was a composer of music and some say the ethereal tone of her work is the foundation for what has come to be known as New Age music.

Centuries later, Lord Alfred Tennyson wrote of death as a diminishing of light and slowing of the "wheels of Being," which could be said to correspond to the chakras, the body's life energy vortexes referred to in Hindu religion.* Certainly light is cross-culturally held to be the essence of spirit or "God," as is reflected in language such as "divine light," the "light of the Holy Spirit" and "enlightenment." The Bible is full of light imagery.

Be near me when my light is low,

When the blood creeps, and the nerves prick

and tingle; and the heart is sick,

And all the wheels of Being slow..."

Lord Alfred Tennyson, In the Valley of Cauteretz, 1847

Here are some quotes from the Bible which seem to relate to Auras:

Now it is high time to awake out of sleep: for now is our salvation nearer than when we believed. The night is far spent, the day is at hand: let us therefore cast off the works of darkness, and let us put on the armor of light."

Corinthians 1, 11

"The Lord is the source of my light and my safety, so whom shall I fear?"

Psalm 26:1

The Aura is often depicted in early Christian art works and Icons such as this one of Jesus from St. Catherine's Monastery in the Sinai from the 6th century AD:

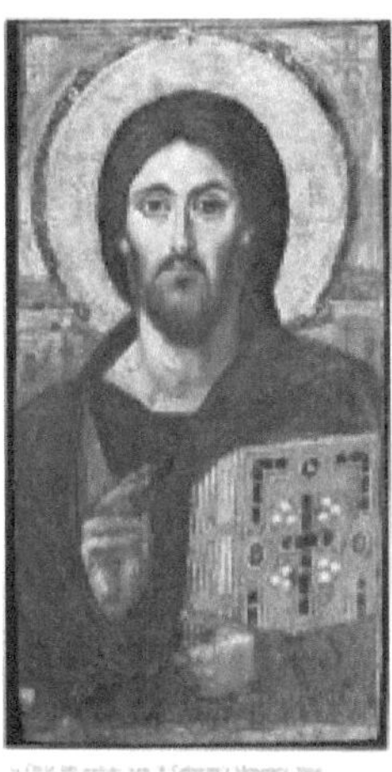

Here is another example of an aura around the head of the Buddha in a statue:

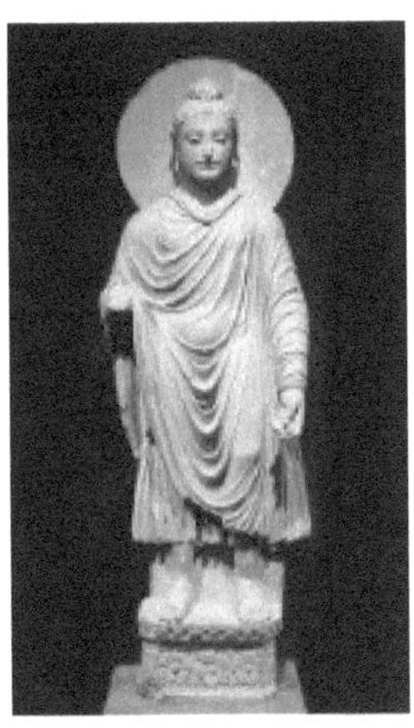

3.0   A Spiritual Basis for Vital Forces

I first read the Yoga Sutras when I was about nineteen, and it has impressed me to this day as a well written exposition for enlightenment and an analytical view of Yoga.

I believe that the Sutras also describes the underlying reality behind all religions and mystical philosophies.

"The Yoga Sutras of Patanjali" was written in four books in the Sanskrit language and is one of the great spiritual works of India.

It is available in print and in many versions on the Internet, and describes the path to enlightenment and attainment of spiritual powers.

The Sutras were written over 2,000 years ago by some estimates.

The Sutras are often described as a scientific exposition in the science of yoga and consists of 4 books of Sutras in Sanskrit which has numerous translations in English.

Each book was written in short sentences of Sanskrit, so many publications of the Yoga Sutras today include the following:

1) The original Sanskrit text

2) The phonetic and exact word translation

3) Turning the previous into and English sentence

4) An exposition on the meaning and details of the Sutra.

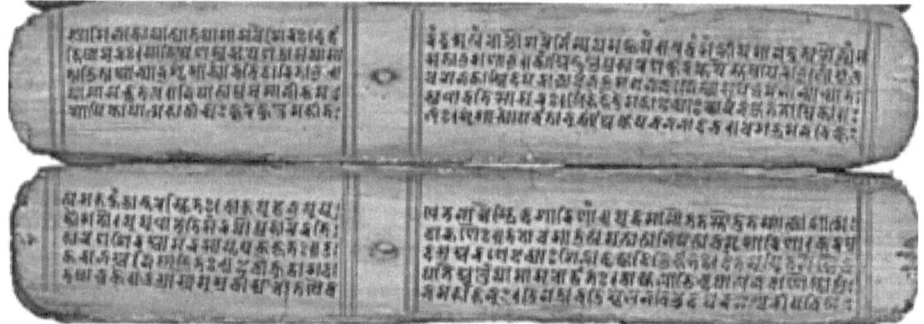

The above picture is of an old wooden slat written in Sanskrit text.

All of the superhuman abilities and powers and more referred to in the Sutras are found in book three.

The goal of the yogic path and the Sutras is enlightenment, however many spiritual powers become side effects of this spiritual process.

Many Sutras describe different abilities or how different abilities can be derived.

This Sutra then provides the basis for the power to exist.

An example is Book 3, Sutra 43 on Teleportation:

The Sanskrit Text and a Phonetic Translation (2)

४३. कायाकाशयो: संबन्धसंयमाल्लघुतूलसमापत्तेश्चा-
काशगमनम् ।

Kāyākāśayoḥ sambandha-saṃyamāt
laghu-tūla-samāpatteś cākāśa-gamanam.

काय (of) the body आकाशयो: (and) space or ether संबन्ध (on) relation संयमात् by performing *Samyama* लघु (with) light (opposite of heavy) तूल cotton down समापत्ते: by coalescence of the mind; by (bringing about) rapport च and आकाश space; sky गमनम् going in; passage through.

43. By performing Samyama on the relation between the body and Akasa and at the same time bringing about coalescence of the mind with light (things like) cotton down (there comes the power of) passage through space.

This passage also infers effects of the mind on physical matter so it also applies to psychokinesis.

****

The vital forces described as the basis for different psychic abilities are all a part of the spiritual structure of consciousness as understood by many enlightened texts and persons down through the age.

The Yoga Sutras, other Vedic scriptures, and more modern organizations like the theosophists all recognize a pretty complex structure to consciousness of which the vital forces we discuss in this book are only a small part.

Theosophy teaches that there are different planes of reality in the universe, such as the physical plane, the astral plane, etc. There are a total of seven planes of existence.

The seven planes of existence, from the highest to the lowest, are:

- Adi Plane
- Anupadaka Plane
- Atman Plane
- Buddhic Plane
- Mental Plane
- Astral Plane
- Physical Plane

Various — and sometimes confusing — naming systems are used in Theosophical literature. Here is a chart.

The Seven Planes of Existence - The Different Naming Systems

1 Atomic 2 3 4 5 6 7	**1**	ADI	MAHAPARANIRVANA (MAHAPARINIRVANA)	DIVINE
1 Atomic 2 3 4 5 6 7	**2**	ANUPADAKA	PARANIRVANA (PARINIRVANA)	MONADIC
1 Atomic 2 3 4 5 6 7	**3**	ATMA	NIRVANA	SPIRITUAL
1 Atomic 2 3 4 5 6 7	**4**	BUDDHI	BUDDHI	INTUITIONAL
1 Atomic 2 3 4 5 6 7	**5**	MENTAL (MANAS)	MENTAL	MENTAL
1 Atomic 2 3 4 5 6 7	**6**	ASTRAL	ASTRAL	ASTRAL
1 Atomic 2 Sub-Atomic 3 Super-Etheral 4 Etheral 5 Gas 6 Liquid 7 Solid	**7**	PHYSICAL	PHYSICAL	PHYSICAL

You will see from this diagram that the chakras, aura, and vital forces channels in our bodies serve multiple levels of energy and consciousness. (3)

The main levels for vital forces energies we will deal with in this book include those on the Physical and Astral planes.

5.0   The Energy Body in Theosophy

The Theosophical Society was officially formed in New York City, United States, in November 1875 by Helena Blavatsky, Henry Steel Olcott, William Quan Judge and others. Its initial objective was the "study and elucidation of Occultism, the Cabala etc."

After a few years Olcott and Blavatsky moved to India and established the International Headquarters at Adyar, in Madras (Chennai). They were also interested in studying Eastern religions, and these were included in the Society's agenda. After several iterations the Society's objectives evolved to be:

1.   To form a nucleus of the universal brotherhood of humanity without distinction of race, creed, sex, caste, or color.

2.   To encourage the study of comparative religion, philosophy, and science.

3.   To investigate the unexplained laws of nature and the powers latent in man.

Theosophists wrote many books on eastern spiritual development, and on the energy body, auras, chakras, thoughtforms and more. I've used some of their material and images from their books because of their great detail and acceptance by the majority of psychics and clairvoyants as being correct.

In the next chapter we will explore the levels of consciousness and the energy body hierarchy per the Yoga Sutras of Patanjali and Theosophical concepts.

6.0   Energy Channels

Learning how to develop vital force energy flows in your body is the first step to achieving successful powers.

The Chinese concept of energy meridians (the points and channels along which energy moves) are used in acupuncture therapy and are another way of looking at the energy flows a body needs.

These and the Indian concept of energy centers (chakras) are all about the way your energy body is designed to stay healthy when energy flows are working properly.

 Above is a diagram of the main acupuncture meridians of the body:

When those flows are interrupted it affects our health and acupuncture can be used to restore this. Needles are used by acupuncturists to stop and start energy moving at key meridian points to help restore the energy body to a proper balance.

**Acupuncture meridians are called many names. These names includes Chinese meridians, energy meridians, and Chi meridians, just to name a few. These meridians carry the life energy that vitalizes all life forms and allows them to grow. Different cultures call this life energy by different names; Chi, subtle energy, life force, Spirit, Prana, and vital energy are all just some of its titles.

Like electricity, this energy is invisible to the human eye. However, some experienced Chinese doctors can feel and trace these pathways of energy with their hands. About

5,000 years ago Chinese doctors mapped these meridian lines. The discovery and understanding of these pathways of energy led to the development of acupuncture to balance Chi.

7.0   The Chakras

The understanding of the chakra systems in our bodies was developed in India thousands of years ago and is now one of the most common metaphysical concepts.

The following diagram is the locations and Hindu names of the most commonly understood chakras:

Many books and traditions discuss details of energy meridians and chakra development so I will not do so here. A short summary of Chakras and their functions follows.

The Figure above shows the chakra centers on the body. These chakras are energy centers where you take in energy to keep your body healthy. The chakras when developed are commonly thought to control spiritual and mental abilities as follows:

Crown Chakra: To be open, to know, intuition, precognition, connection   with infinite intelligence, to have faith and connection with God

Below is a picture of the crown chakra as seen psychically. It is also often known as the thousand petal lotus:

3rd eye Chakra: Clairvoyance, psychic reading, to have vision or insight, photographic memory and telekinesis

Throat Chakra: Communication center, telepathy, clairaudience, inner   voice and tone healing

Heart Chakra: To be in affinity with, to be at one with, to connect with, compassion and unconditional love.

Here is another psychic picture of the heart chakra:

Solar Plexus Chakra: Astral projection, to be empowered, to manifest, to be in control of yourself, psychic healing and levitation

Sacrum/Feeling Chakra: Clairsentience, emotional feelings, balance of   male and female energies

Root Chakra: Grounding, realizing, letting go, and surviving

8.0　　The Aura, and it's Colors and Patterns

The human aura has been illustrated many different ways since we really don't have any good photographic techniques to show how it looks. Here are a few illustrations which are close to my own observations:

The above two images are the closest I could find to what the aura looks like. It is a gaseous cloud emanating and surrounding the individual, with different densities and colors around the chakras.

This image below shows a good illustration of what the different aura layers can represent:

Aura colors may be interpreted differently, but here are some common meanings of colors you might see in the human Aura:

RED AURA COLOR MEANING: Relates to the physical body, hart or circulation. The densest color, it creates the most friction. Friction attracts or repels; money worries or obsessions; anger or unforgiveness; anxiety or nervousness

Deep Red: Grounded, realistic, active, strong will-power, survival-oriented.

Muddied red: Anger (repelling)

Clear red: Powerful, energetic, competitive, sexual, passionate

Pink-bright and light: Loving, tender, sensitive, sensual, artistic, affection, purity, compassion; new or revived romantic relationship. Can indicate clairaudience.

Dark and murky pink: Immature and/or dishonest nature

Orange Red: Confidence, creative power

In a good, bright and pure state, red energy can serve as a healthy ego.

ORANGE AURA COLOR: Relates to reproductive organs and emotions. The color of vitality, vigor, good health and excitement. Lots of energy and stamina, creative, productive, adventurous, courageous, outgoing social nature; currently experiencing stress related to appetites and addictions;

Orange-Yellow: Creative, intelligent, detail oriented, perfectionist, scientific.

YELLOW AURA COLOR MEANING: Relates to the spleen and life energy. It is the color of awakening, inspiration, intelligence and action shared, creative, playful, optimistic, easy-going.

Light or pale yellow: Emerging psychic and spiritual awareness; optimism and hopefulness; positive excitement about new ideas.

Bright lemon-yellow: Struggling to maintain power and control in a personal or business relationship; fear of losing control, prestige, respect, and/or power.

Clear gold metallic, shiny and bright: Spiritual energy and power activated and awakened; an inspired person.

Dark brownish yellow or gold: A student, or one who is straining at studying; overly analytical to the point of feeling fatigued or stressed; trying to make up for "lost time" by learning everything all at once.

GREEN AURA COLOR MEANING: Relates to heart and lungs. It is a very comfortable, healthy color of nature. When seen in the aura this usually represents growth and balance, and most of all, something that leads to change. Love of people, animals, nature; teacher; social

Bright emerald green: A healer, also a love-centered person

Yellow-Green: Creative with heart, communicative

Dark or muddy forest green: Jealousy, resentment, feeling like a victim of the world; blaming self or others; insecurity and low self-esteem; lack of understanding personal responsibility; sensitive to perceived criticism

Turquoise: Relates to the immune system. Sensitive, compassionate, healer, therapist.

BLU AURA COLOR MEANING: Relates to the throat, thyroid. Cool, calm, and collected. Caring, loving, love to help others, sensitive, intuitive.

Soft blue: Peacefulness, clarity and communication; truthful; intuitive

Bright royal blue: Clairvoyant; highly spiritual nature; generous; on the right path; new opportunities are coming

Dark or muddy blue: Fear of the future; fear of self-expression; fear of facing or speaking the truth

INDIGO AURA COLOR MEANING: Relates to the third eye, visual and pituitary gland. Intuitive, sensitive, deep feeling.

VIOLET AURA COLOR MEANING: Relates to crown, pineal gland and nervous system. The most sensitive and wisest of colors. This is the intuitive color in the aura, and reveals psychic power of attunement with self. Intuitive, visionary, futuristic, idealistic, artistic, magical.

LAVENDER AURA COLOR MEANING: Imagination, visionary, daydreamer, etheric.

SILVER AURA COLOR MEANING: This is the color of abundance, both spiritual and physical. Lots of bright silver can reflect to plenty of money, and/or awakening of the cosmic mind.

Bright metallic silver: Receptive to new ideas; intuitive; nurturing

Dark and muddy gray: Residue of fear is accumulating in the body, with a potential for health problems, especially if gray clusters seen in specific areas of the body

GOLD AURA COLOR MEANING: The color of enlightenment and divine protection. When seen within the aura, it says that the person is being guided by their highest good. It is divine guidance. Protection, wisdom, inner knowledge, spiritual mind, intuitive thinker.

BLACK AURA COLOR MEANING: Draws or pulls energy to it and in so doing, transforms it. It captures light and consumes it. Usually indicates long-term unforgiveness (toward others or another) collected in a specific area of the body, which can lead to health problems; also, entities within a person's aura, chakras, or body; past life hurts; unreleased grief from abortions if it appears in the ovaries

WHITE AURA COLOR MEANING: Reflects other energy. A pure state of light. Often represents a new, not yet designated energy in the aura. Spiritual, etheric and nonphysical qualities, transcendent, higher dimensions. Purity and truth; angelic qualities.

White sparkles or flashes of white light: angels are nearby; can indicate that the person is pregnant or will be soon

EARTH AURA COLORS: Soil, wood, mineral, plant. These colors display a love of the Earth, of being grounded and is seen in those who live and work on the outdoors....construction, farming, etc. These colors are important and are a good sign.

RAINBOWS: Rainbow-colored stripes, sticking out like sunbeams from the hand, head or body: A Reiki healer, or a star person (someone who is in the first incarnation on Earth)

PASTELS: A sensitive blend of light and color, more so than basic colors. Shows sensitivity and a need for serenity.

DIRTY BROWN OVERLAY: Holding on to energies. Insecurity.

DIRTY GRAY OVERLY: Blocking energies. Guardedness.

9.0 Energy Body Evidence

(Transcript of Video)

Okay we're going to talk about the energy body-the vital body. There's a lot of different words for it the-vital life force-and I'm going to take a different approach here a little more Socratic rather than just talking about it. Because I think most of you are pretty familiar with the concept and just reviewing that concept you know we think it's the force that enlivens us.

But let me ask you guys what evidence have you had in your lives about the energy body really existing. Could I hear a couple people talk about why they think they have an energy body? But somebody should speak up because it's not something that science observes. Yeah go ahead.

Okay so you see the auras-that's good-that's to know if you see something. It's usually good-yes-be between people. Cool it has mine the kind of connections between people and you saw that after you came back.

Anybody else? Go ahead Lynn-I was in a class with a Fung Shui master and she rubbed hands together and then holding like this and you could feel the energy course going between them. Yeah that's a good way to do it. I'm working with biofeedback and of course lead biofeedback equipment will read the energy body and I find it especially worked with animals. And with anything up at my dog that she had a dislocated shoulder that couldn't figure out. People's x-ray and she just recently had a big infection on her leg that went right into her bone and that didn't know what it was from. So Joseph and all your training did you have any dramatic experiences with the energy body that you could share. I guess you have called the energy body in yoga practice when you connect with a master of yoga which usually is a spiritual teacher. A spiritual master rather than just the hatha yoga type of tradition. If you have a master yogi and you connect with them and do practices under their supervision etc then I would be blessed one time doing.

I was doing every day milk and fruit and I was doing my in dental practices and I was able to dislocate from my body and travel outside of my physical body. You know you can see your body-you know it's there and you're off somewhere else. It is commonly called astral body-yeah I think those people would go there.

And a lot of traditions talk about multiple levels of the energy body to up to the Atman. Theosophists and a lot of yogic traditions talk about that so there seems to be a lot of let's call it subjective evidence from our experience. That the energy body exists and that's a big reason we're talking about it. I'm sure you've all seen aura pictures and you know what I'm not going to even go into that except to say different people say different chakras mean different things. But I think there's common agreement that there's also common agreement that there are energy meridians. And everybody of course we know about the Chinese and their acupuncture which was thousands of years old that helps manipulate the energy pathways in your body. So there's a lot of people over a long period of time who both see the energy body have had experiences with the energy body.

Experiences are between people with the energy body so we were pretty confident that it exists and we talked about that. The Chinese meridians-I'm going to do a couple short exercises with you one is a Qigong exercise and you might want to stand up because I'm sure you're sick of sitting. A

And then this quite Qigong related to but a little different than Tai Chi. In Qigong you do things to manipulate the energy forces and one of the exercises which the instructor claimed was a secret exercise-but I'll share it with you because you didn't swear me to secrecy. Is that what we're going to do here so just stand calmly with your hands down here at your sides and what I want you to imagine is in your body cavity. You can probably want to close your eyes and your body cavity you want to imagine that your vital forces are going to be rolling indifferent directions.

Okay there's three different axes we're going to move our energy forces in. First of all I want you to imagine inside your body your vital forces are moving from the top down the front and up inside the back and feel for a while the energy flowing inside your body cavity. The vital force flowing down inside-through your organs through you're your abdomen and then back up back up and near your back and around. Okay the next flow and these are just short this is something you could practice for15 or 20 minutes every day.

Next flow we're going to talk about we're going to have going from left to right in the circle clockwise so imagine the energy in your torso around the central like you've got a central pole in the middle of you-is going to go around this pole from your left side going around to the right in front and then around to the back. Over from the right to left and at the energy inside your body cavity is flowing and you can feel the energy moving back around to the front.

Now to the right to the back and then to the left-okay and one more axis so we've done top down and around they've done left right and actually I think I covered all the sides so that's the idea. That's something you can carry on-do that five or ten minutes a day and the choice the Qigong instructor claimed that would help vital moves in the vital center for energy forces among your organs and that that would be very helpful.

So that's just one little exercise. Okay we're done with that-you can sit down. Okay how many people have done exercises to be able to see auras-see the human aura? Okay seeing the human aura is not difficult it just takes the right way of focusing. Now like many things-some people have more of a natural ability than others. Like my son-he probably doesn't want me to say but he can see floors in color and whereas I don't see the color I see more shadows.

But here's a little exercise that I found I can do like when I'm sitting in a classroom-when I'm getting bored. Hopefully that's not the case right now but that I would do this and what you do is just sit-there look at me with a background behind me. It helps to have a solid background of some in front it. Focus your eyes-look straight on at me but de focus your eyes okay-and as you focus your eyes kind of use your peripheral vision. If you use your peripheral vision then when your eyes are relaxed and be focused you might start to see a haze around me. Around more maybe more around my head because I'm more energized there-but it may be out to a distance of a couple inches. That's the typical light haze of the inner aura and you just have to let your eyes relax to do it.

When you when you relax you can see that glow around people and you can also see it around objects, and after you do it enough times it becomes second nature. So you can see-many people can see that-can you see that. Okay it's not hard to see you just have to not try to look. You have to relax and let your eyes see it and use your peripheral vision to do it.

Okay-yes you know usually when you start doing it you don't see the colors and it's like being an athlete. Different people have different abilities but through practice-and many of these techniques as you practice it-you will learn more. You will learn to see more detail and more colors. For instance I don't see chakras too well. Other people I know including my son see chakras in detail, and can see all the details swirling and stuff like that.

And again I think it's a combination of practice and innate ability but we can all-I think most of us can learn to see the basic or just by a little practice.

How many of you heard of Kirlian photography. Okay-most of you it was most popular in the 70s when I was in college. I was actually doing some research on it and what it was all about was trying to use a photographic technique involving high frequency high energy discharges from a Tesla coil for different objects-Often fingers.

But it could be plants and things directly on photographic film. And then you would process the film after it was exposed. This way you would get some really interesting discharge patterns. The claim was that the discharge patterns would show different emotional states. It's hard to verify these things but I had some interesting experience with it one of these are some of my pictures are here-the damaged leaf-this is where i puta cut and leave and you can see there's a little red area there why red for a damaged area? I don't know but I thought it was pretty interesting other claims were that different emotions would show in specific colors-that red could be anger, and in other colors like white-they could represent love or spiritual feelings. So I would do some experiments with people to think different emotions while we were generating these Kirlian discharge patterns. And the affects you got were real interesting. Now as a scientist I won't claim that it's absolute evidence of emotions in your aura but I will say it was pretty interesting. It's very hard to pin down because there's a lot of different variables involved but it's probably the closest we've come to being able to measure this in a scientific manner. I'll be honest this is like 35 years ago so I don't remember exactly. I didn't caption these slides unfortunately I don't remember exactly what the thought was. This one I recall was more of an anger emotion here --and I mean I never thought I would be using these slides for anything so I didn't caption them at the time. But you did one of the things that was interesting as you would get different patterns from different emotions that was the cool thing.

10.0 Chakra Energy Flows

(Transcript of Video)

All right I'm going to do a more intense energy exercise. It's somewhat similar to what Sophia did this morning but it's going to be more intense. And I want to give you some history of this. When I was nineteen in engineering school I had a mentor. His name was Sam Lentine. He since passed on-he was a middle-aged guy who was a blind highly psychic physicist. Okay-an interesting combination and he taught me this exercise. The beginning of this exercise which I've since elaborated in the first relaxation meditation course I ever took. And it's all about learning how to take in energy into your crown chakra and manipulate it through the other energy centers of your body. And what I found is after doing it a few times it became very intense and I could actually feel a real heat inside of me-and after I'd been doing this a while probably a number of months it started to happen spontaneously and in all that time which must be about 30 plus years now I still have a lot of instances when spontaneously I'll start having huge amounts of energy come in through my crown.

And then other parts of my body may be also take in energy-now this exercise if you've never done anything like this once you start to feel the effects of it. You may start to question it in terms of how you know whether it's going to damage you but I don't think so. It's a good exercise-it's just manipulation of body force or energy force rather and you really will feel an intense feeling-maybe not the first time but if you keep doing it several times I think that will come. And what it does is it that brings that life force in to help strengthen you.

One of the things I found happens a lot with me is it would come in and strengthen my heart. I would actually feel it coming in. If you don't know if you've ever felt like-you had like totally no energy and you felt like you're just totally blah in the chest-well I would do this when I felt that way and I just felt totally vital inside and alive again.

Now that you're relaxed I want you to start visualizing a cone coming down from infinity with a point of it intersecting into the top of your head. The top of your head is with a thousand pedal lotuses the crown chakra. The place of God's intersection with you-with your spirit as you feel this cone in the top of your head you want to feel the energy of that God force coming down and as it comes down its brilliant white.

And it gets more compressed as it gets and this comes down-it's flowing into the top of your head. This is power, this is energy, this is God's force coming into the top of your head and it's going to start coming into you. As you breathe in you'll feel it flow into you. Breathe out relax, breathe in, you feel it flow into you more intensely as it starts coming down inside your head. This energy first activates your third eye and your third eye-it starts opening and as it opens more energy is coming in through it and the result of two energies mixed together-and travel down further into your neck. Again breathe in, and visualize that white fire-brilliant white energy coming into your head traveling down now to your throat. Your Throat Chakra's opening-as it opens you also feel it's swirling and energy coming in from there too. The energy continues to come down to you and it's getting more intense. The power of it is increasing and this is the vital force that enlightens you. Now it's travelling down your neck and you can feel it coming into your heart. And it fills it up to overflowing again.

Breathe in and you should start to feel heat-just start to feel a fire coming in down from your head through your neck-into your chest as you feel that you also feel your heart opening and with your heart opening you feel unconditional love. You'll know it when you feel it. It's a powerful experience of God's love for everyone and everything. Now the energy is getting denser. It's flowing down-and from your head, your neck, into your chest.

Now further you're sacrum-the navel and that you feel it opening. As you feel it opening you feel energy flowing in there. You feel the power flowing in there. Continue to breathe in-energy comes in through the top and through the other opening points that you've made. As you breathe out its just peaceful relaxation now we continue when we go further down to the root chakra. The root chakra-you feel that opening-as that's opening you feel intensity of fire there. You have the Kundalini the earth energy coming at your base is locked into the earth. And you feel the energy coming up through the base of your spine mixing with the energy from the crown and they will start heading back up your spine.

You can imagine that you've got a white intense light traveling up your spine and that light travels up your spine and it keeps going up and up. You breathe in again the energy comes down through your crown now in through the other chakras and passes through your heart all the way down to your root. And your energy mixes with energy from the ground and fire comes back up through your spine all the way up behind your chest now into the base of your head. And mixes there so now we have a flow of energy through the major centers of your body front and back.

Let's do this again-so you can feel it more intensely. Okay-again you have the point of the cone coming down into your head. You can now feel that there's a flow like a waterfall a brilliant light healing God's energy coming into you. Coming down through your head coming down and through your neck opening the Centers of the navel-coming down into your heart opening your heart center.

Travelling further down traveling down to the belly and then back to down to the root. Mixing with the fire from the earth fire that comes back up your spine back-into your head. Once you just continue to feel that cycle for a couple more minutes and know that each time you do this it will be more intense and they will be vitalize your system. It will create more synchronicity between your spirit your energy in your body because this is the energy from God that feeds your energy body that feeds your physical body. This will make you healthier and more vital and able to connect to oneness. Okay-so when you're ready you can slowly open your eyes. Okay-thank you anybody feel anything? Again it can be a very intense feeling once it really starts to happen. That's why I like this and then it can happen spontaneously so it's one of my favorite exercises.

11.0 The Emerald Tablets

(Video Transcript)

Hello and welcome to this presentation about body polarity and how that affects your relationship with immortality or longevity. This is from the Emerald Tablets by Thoth the Atlantean. An interesting metaphysical book from many years ago according to the ancient artifact referred to as the Emerald Tablet.

It was supposedly written by Thoth the Atlantean. It states you know that the body when in perfect balance may never be touched by the finger of death. When you were in balanced equilibrium you shall live on in time and not taste of death. You have a balanced completion existing because of the balance poles of the body and know that the secret of life in heaven is a secret of restoring the balance of the poles so that all that has existed has form and is living because of the spirit of life.

And it's poles you can also know that the Earth's heart is a balance of all things that exist and have being on its face the source of your spirit is drawn from Earth's heart. And your body is formed as one with the earth and when you learn to hold your balance you will draw on the balance of the Earth so if you're truly one with the Earth your form will not be based on that. So what does all this mean? It continues so the secret of holding your form is as follows according to the Emerald Tablet. One hour each day point your head towards the positive pole or North of the Earth while your head is placed in the northward direction.

Hold your consciousness in the center of the chest to the top of your head. Next for one hour each day point your head towards the negative pole or South of the Earth when you're pointing your head in the South direction. Hold in your consciousness in the center of your chest to the bottom of the feet again. Do this visualization exercise every day now when you look at this diagram you'll see that the four traditional elements of the ancients: Air, Fire, Water, and Earth, are all related to the different parts of your body. And this is the concept behind balance and polarity and how it affects your longevity according to the ancients.

Another set of sayings-hold yourself in balance every seven minutes and your balance will retain the whole of its strength. If you look and feel old the body will freshen your strength-will become as a youth. This is a secret known to the Masters by which they hold off the finger of death. Neglect not to follow the path of thought showing for when you have passed beyond your years of two hundred. To neglect it will mean the coming of death. Hear my words and follow a path way-keep your balance and live on in life. Now we talk about mastering eternal time according to the Emerald Tablets. Eternal time can be mastered it states that we should learn the secret that is the master of time. This skill will allow you to remember the lives of the past-a great secret yet easy to master. Which will give you the mastery of when you feel death is fast approaching through the following fear not and know that you are a master of death. Relax the body with no tension. Place in your heart the flame of your soul swiftly sweep it to the seat of the triangle

Hold for a moment then move to between the eyebrows. This is the place between your eyebrows-the place where the memory of life must hold sway again. Instructions for visualization next hold the flame of the soul here in your brain seat until the fingers of death grasp your soul. And as you pass through the staff of transition slowly the memories of life shall pass – then shall the past be as one with the present then shall the memory of all be retained. You will be forever be free from regression. That things of the past shall live in today with this knowledge you will be one of the Masters of mystery. Conquerors of death and masters of life thank you for listening again. These are the principles of Thoth the Immortal from ancient times. Make of them what you will by now.

12.0 Cell Regeneration Exercise

Okay this is one of my favorite exercises. I'm not going to say that I originated it although I was elaborating it. I actually saw that parts of this from a book called "Star Signs" but Linda Goodman used to know her. Okay so she's passed on but she had some really interesting thoughts. The exercise we're going to go through in a minute is where if you imagine the spiral is the life of yourself from birth, the cells in your body the center circle is when the cell was born the star is the age of your cells exist today.

What we're going to do is we're going to use this visualization technique to travel back to an earlier point in your cells life and we're going to do this throughout the body. And the idea is where as a clock goes clockwise as time progresses we're going to use counter clockwise. I did say clockwise-right clockwise. Spiral counterclockwise as a visualization to show that we're going backwards in time. So I'd like you at all to sit down and prepare yourself for a few minutes-to get in a very relaxed state and then we're going to go through this.

I'd also like to mention before we get started is that I did this one night the first time I tried it and I did it for about half an hour and I felt like it was having a really good effect. But I didn't know of the things that were said in that book "Star Signs" was that after you've done this exercise for some time it didn't say the first time but after you've done it and it was starting to take effect that other people or yourself might notice a smell of like leather old shoes and that the idea was that as toxins are released from your cells that creates some odor which you can take a shower or cover up some odor that other people can notice. But that's okay if you're getting younger right.

Okay-all right so anyway the next morning the next morning I'm taking my son to school and my son being a regular kid who doesn't like to shower unless he's forced to doesn't ever complain about my smell. And he says "Dad you smell today". I said what the heck are you talking about? "You smell like leather or something". Okay that's a really interesting comment.

Oh-so anyway okay so let's close our eyes let's get relaxed. Breathe for a minute or two get centered because these visualization exercises are most effective the more centered that you are. That's the whole reason we work on being centered before we get into these things. Okay I'd like you to pick a physical age that you want your body to revert to. An age where you felt the healthiest, the most, where you may be the happiest-whatever age that is that you want to be going forward. Now we're going to start and work in different parts of our body. I want you to go into your left foot. I want you to imagine your vision is expanding down to the microscopic level. The microscopic level where you can actually see cells up close-where you go into a cell. Just pick any one cell and you're inside that cell, and you're merging with it you're-merging with its consciousness you're feeling it. You're one with the cell and the age of the cell. You can kind of feel how old that cell is and that now you have determined that your age of the cell is going backwards that the health of the cell is becoming more vital-more alive. It's going back to the age that you've chosen and as it becomes more vital the processes heat up any accumulated waste-flows out of the cell.

Now expand that viewpoint so you're looking at fifty or a hundred cells still living in your foot-maybe within your big toe. Now you expand your view point. You see the energy from that one permeating into the others and that will be because there is a will involved here will not only of you at a body level but the will of the individual cell. And as you as that will permeates and that energy permeates those other cells also start to unwind and you can actually see in your mind's eye a spiral going backwards counterclockwise of the time that each cell is going backwards in time.

It's reverting to an earlier state of being. You may start to feel a tingling in that area. Now start expanding your vision more so that you're feeling the toes in your foot-toes in your left foot and that this reverse spiral is reverse aging-is expanding within those cells. That they're becoming more vital more alive. They're throwing off old ways the telomeres are becoming longer in the DNA. That they're becoming more alive and you're may start to feel something. You're following me if you start to feel tingling there. Now you can imagine not only the spirals inside of each cell as they revert but a spiral around that part of your foot and a macro spiral-it's going that swirling around your foot above your toes and below and above. And below again counterclockwise. And I want you to imagine this is a reverse spiral. The larger level is starting to move up your toes to your foot, to your heel, and as it does the same thing is occurring at a microscopic level inside of each cell because the energy the using of each cell-the reverse aging is in your foot.

That sensation is becoming more powerful and we go up into the calf up to the knee. We have a large spiral around our leg reversing as each cell individually. I's catching on to the same process just like the consciousness of the cells are talking to each other-so they're working at a microscopic level as you are working at a macroscopic level.

Reversal is continuing up your thigh to the top of your leg and you can feel that it's happening. You can feel that the cells are going back to a younger age. You actually feel that they are a younger age. You can feel like how did that part of your body feel when you were that age-was there more muscle? was it more supple? Imagine the state that your body was in from the cellular level-the macroscopic level for your left leg.

Now let's start and do the same thing on the right leg. Start down in the toes at a cellular level-that we see the spiral going around our toes. A reverse spiral that each cell has its own spiral as its anti-aging-it's caught the feeling too-caught the consciousness from the other leg. Now we travel up the foot there's a larger spiral growing and as we're doing this we're feeling a greater power and intensity of this progressing in our body. We go up-go up our foot includes the heel. Start to go up our leg spiral around our leg up to our knee and now our thigh all the way up to the top of our leg and again the consciousness is working at an individual cellular level where it's communicating this. Is the way we're going to be this is the order as well as at the larger level of visualizing how your right leg was at that earlier time how it felt. Okay. Now we're going to start traveling up the trunk of the body from your bottom going up your abdomen-feel the spiral around you.

It's like a reverse galaxy with you in the center of it spiraling backwards in time. You can actually feel the energy and the spiraling backwards in time going up your abdomen. The spiral is around the outside of your body and penetrates into the cells and as that's doing it each cell inside it's catching on each cell. Understanding this is the way it must be-this is the new life-this is the vitality reverting to that earlier age traveling up your chest through your liver, your lungs, your heart, Your bodies are reverting even your skin-you're visualizing how your skin cells are reverting to that earlier age or their tightening.

We're looking more supple-spots are disappearing. Everything about your skin is becoming younger. Travelling up your chest now-up under your upper chest and inside your chest all the cells from your bones, your muscles, your organs. All tissue are now on board with us. They are now feeling like there at this earlier age. Imagine again the reverse spirals inside of each cell-millions of billions of them all part of this consciousness to revert to the earlier age. To become the earlier age you're not just reverting but your cells are feeling that they are part of that earlier age. They are the earlier age of your body traveling up now to your neck.

Now let's stop and do each arm-to the left arm feel this whole spiral travelling from the tips of your fingers up your hand to your wrist. Through your forearm again the reverse spiral inside and outside up your left arm-all the way to the shoulder. Now the right arm-the fingertips feel and pick the penetrating interpenetrating all your cells of your hand-your right wrist. The forearm-now the upper arm up to the shoulder.

Now we'll continue going up your neck-can spiral around you outside of your neck interpenetrating your cells as each cell becomes part of this. One conscious effort into your head. All parts of your head-your teeth are growing new roots-any problems you've had with your sinuses are reverting to an earlier age. You're hearing is renewing as it feels inside. Revert to that earlier age become the earlier you and your brain. Same thing earlier health up to the top of your head. Now at this point you are whole. You should start to be feeling an energization that everything is reverting to that earlier age.

Everything is at that earlier age and outside of you-the energy spiral is spiraling around all your limbs and your entire body. And that energy is taking your energy field back to that earlier age too. You feel more youthful, you feel you were that age, you are that age your body. Just has to catch up with the energy because it won't happen instantly but it happens now. The cells have a pattern to follow. They have a blueprint they now understand what they need to become, and that's more youthful taking you back to that earlier age. Okay, so just feel that for a minute little sensations inside your body down to the cell level. Any sensations of tingling or energy as you do this and you have complete power because your body is conscious. Your energy field is conscious and you've now given it a new direction.

You've given it the direction of what you want your body to be you've told it that's what you are to become. Okay, now you can slowly open your eyes. Okay so did anybody you feel anything? Okay this is something you probably want to do every day. You do it whenever you're meditating or you're just lying there getting ready to go to bed. I've been feeling better. I am 25 mentally-I don't know if you see it yet.

13.0 Sacred Fire

(Video Transcript)

Okay, the Sacred Fire visualization is an ancient exercise. The books unveiled mysteries and magic presence talk about it. Many people called it secret exercise. It's not that complex-but it's very powerful and it's another one of these exercises that we're going to do from a meditative state.

Talks about a pillar of white fire penetrating your being. We're going to go through that and when you do this you should feel something. It's amazing-I put it on a par with the cell regeneration exercise which is also one of my favorites.

Close your eyes do some deep breathing or relax however you want to do it-to get centered you want to center yourself. The center of your head and your pineal gland-the traditional location of the spirit or soul. I want you to imagine that there's a bright white pillar of fire coming down-surrounding you-and also there's a bright light like a flame in the center of your head. This flame is going to get brighter, and brighter, and brighter. Started going to get brighter and as it gets brighter it expands. This is the pure white fire of God's spirit expanding into your head-interpenetrating your cells-travelling down your neck into your chest this bright light starting to fill you with purity and health. The bright white light travels down your torso, into your arms-your legs and this keeps going on and getting more intense until you imagine yourself a vessel of white light.

This white light is so intense it's like staring at the Sun and even brighter. Now this light is fully penetrating you. It starts expanding beyond the surface of your body first-it's a few inches beyond the surface of your body. Now it expands further out to several feet within that pillar of white light that we started with and the pillar of white light expands further out to ten feet from you. Now you're becoming the center of a sphere of light and consciousness and this light is as bright as the Sun.

I want you to feel and visualize this power is becoming more intense within and outside your body. And more intense now something interesting happens. You start seeing in your head again the light is washing away and dissolving impurities that are unhealthy. Any diseased cells are being washed away and will be expelled from the body. You may sense tiny black areas throughout your head and going into your body within the white light and the white light surrounds and penetrates those areas and dissolves them.

Purifying your body-burning these areas clean for this incredible power-this infinite power of spirit-any impurities or unhealthy cells are being washed away and will be expelled from your body and as things are washed away and expelled any black spots disappear.

And it becomes pure white light again. And you want to travel from your head down from your neck into your chest-and as you're doing this as your kind of imagining a plane, a flat, surface traveling down-penetrating these areas. All of these diseased or bad areas are being washed away and all it's being left and its wake is pure white energy. Immortalizing energy down into your chest, your abdomen, your bottom all the way down your legs to your feet. So now you see your body-you see it inside this pillar of fire. But it's more than fire it's brilliant white light brighter than the Sun. The type of light that's blinding and within that your body is purified. The cells are purified and immortalized because now that now that they're pure they can stay in synchronization with your spirit and the energy feeds them and makes them healthy and keeps them whole. Keep doing this for another minute or two again going back and forth through different parts of your body. Visualizing the white light washing away any impurities-dissolving any impurities and the intensity increasing until you are ultimately a being of light-an ascended being of bright white light.

14.0 Qigong Visualization Video

(Video Transcript)

Hello this is Marty Ettington and in this section of the course we're going to talk about Qigong. Qigong is an ancient Chinese discipline which helps people integrate the energy flows in their body. Get them moving better-it's also often taught with Tai Chi which is also about movement for increasing energy flows. One of the unique things about Qigong is it does have exercises specifically related to longevity.

The Chinese who developed Qigong believed that longevity has to do with the energy center in your lower abdomen-about a thumb below your navel and several inches back in the middle of your abdomen in conjunction with activations for the root chakra at the base of your spine. So what I'm going to do with you in this video is a short visualization exercise which you should practice every day to help build the vitality and life force inside your lower body.

Ready-I'm going to close my eyes as I'd like you to do so and I want you to visualize you're getting relaxed. Go through whatever relaxation technique you do and have your consciousness moved down to your lower abdomen. Visualize inside of your body about thumb below your navel two or three inches in and there's a bright ball of energy there that is your vitality energy center. This energy center is extremely bright-you feel it like a little star and you love it and its part of your body's consciousness which you're connecting with.

This energy star contains your long-term vitality in your abdomen. I want you to realize that this is an important center for the body to keep the body vital, and you will feel this energy center growing every day. You will feel energy coming into your body in your navel area every day to vitalize this energy center. Continue to feel this-now I want you to take your mind to the base of your spine, which is where the root chakra is. The root chakra is what draws energy from the ground and also vitalizes energy distribution through your spine and other energy pathways in your body. A bright globe of energy at the base of your spine. Again it's like another star-this energy center is bright and glowing brighter, and you feel the energy coming up from the ground. Its heat as it comes up it pulses through the base of your spine and up your spine you feel this light from the ground coming up through the base of your spine.

Pulsing up your spine higher and higher and the energy is distributing through the rest of your body. Now you feel a connection between the two energy centers-a connection between the root chakra at the base of your spine and the energy center in your abdomen. The two are communicating passing energy back and forth and strengthening each other. Again go to visualize the energy center in your abdomen-feel it bright. You feel vitality life force is building their life force which vitalizes your entire body and then threw the connection you feel the connection to your root chakra and the bright ball of energy. Your root chakra is vitalizing the bringing of energy into your body. And it's also distributing it to the energy center in your abdomen.

You can feel the energy coming in and going into that vitality energy center. You can open your eyes now this is something you should do for about ten minutes twice a day and as you do it over a week or two you will start to feel more vitality there. And you might even feel the energy coming into your insides again. There's a lot of different types of energy exercises you can do with vital forces in your body and this is a good one to practice. Thank you

15.0 Summary

I hope you enjoyed this book about the Energy Body.

Some adept practitioners believe that manipulating the vital forces can make us immortal. The Masters of Qigong in particular believe this.

There is no doubt to me that my ability to take in vital forces energies through my Crown Chakra and Heart Chakra have made incredible differences in my life.

Those two Chakras are the ones which I've had the most experiences with, but the other chakras are important too and can also result in powerful experiences.

I strongly recommend learning how to open these chakras and the rest of them because it will help your health, longevity, and general experiences with life to a wonderful extent.